# INTRO DUCTION

I'm going to keep this brief, because we have a LOT of names to cover here.

I wrote this book because it was long overdue. I, like millions of you, have a 20-year headache from constantly rolling my eyes at the stupid names people started giving their children over the past generation. This includes both stupid names, and stupid spellings of otherwise non-stupid names. There is a lot of material here. A LOT.

Nothing is this book is made up. All of the names herein are real names that have really been given to real children. Many were plucked off parenting and baby websites. Others are my friends' children. Still more are my actual blood relatives. All were given to their children by dickhead parents who think they're cute or creative or original or novel or trailblazing or sophisticated.

They are none of these things. They are actually just dickheads who love the smell of their own farts and the sound of their own voices. Their desperate need for others to tell them how creative and thoughtful and special they are far outweighs any concern for whether the small human they're raising will actually be happy that they're named after such things as — including but not limited to — a season, a country, a feeling, a poem, a sound, an adjective, an alcoholic beverage, or a sex act. (Yeah. Keep reading. They're all here.)

The psychological community has a special term for these people, and that term is "dickhead."

And although they deserve it, you can't scream at these parents or shake them or kick them or punch them or even loudly ridicule them. First of all, there are too many of them, so you could never get the job done in full. Second, it would make you look like a giant insensitive asshole. You know what they say: nobody wants to hear that they have an ugly baby. Or, in this case, a baby with a really, really fucking stupid name.

So I offer my services to you herein. I'll be your giant insensitive asshole through which you vent your irritation at parents who name their kids after booze, cities, bands, musical genres, cars, sunglasses, building materials, and did I mention, booze? And my personal favorites, the ones who like a name that's actually a name, but can't stomach spelling it in a way that doesn't confuse the living shit out of everyone or shatter the rules of grammar, spelling and punctuation.

Over the next 100 or so pages, I've done all the ridiculing we need on behalf of you and the rest of us who are tired of not being able to say, spell or pronounce ¾ of the students' names at our kids' schools. My comments are vile, belittling and downright unfriendly.

I apologize for nothing.

Yours very truly,
Johnny Dongle

# 1
# Breckstin

**Pop Quiz: What is a Breckstin?**

**(A)** A dangerous chemical byproduct of the ore-smelting process

**(B)** A shampoo that gives your hair extra body and that salon shine!

**(C)** The dumbest fucking name ever given to a child

I know what you're thinking, "Out of all the fucked-up names I've heard of that stupid modern parents are inventing for their kids, I've never heard anyone actually name their kid something as stupid as Breckstin. Can't be true." Right?

Wrongsies! Breckstin is the actual name of at least one actual kid. I feel sorry for Breckstin. No one will ever know how to spell her name, and people will always lie to her about how beautiful her name is. And no one will ever tell her parents what utter fucking dipshits they are for saddling their kid with a name that ridiculous. Until now, anyway.

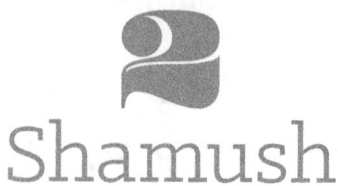

# Shamush

No, I did not misspell "Seamus." The fucking dude's name is Shamush. It's like an Eskimo fucked an orca, and this was the hybrid piece-of-shit name they came up with.

I don't know how the parents pronounce this name — I just read it somewhere. I would guardedly assume it's pronounced like it's spelled, so that every time the parents yell out for the little feller, it sounds like the noise that's made when someone steps on a junebug.

Of course, as stupid as his parents obviously are, it's probably pronounced like Shay-mus...or even Shay-moose. Or, more likely, his parents are probably too fucked up on meth and kerosene to even say his name.

The good news is, I am certain that a kid with parents irresponsible enough to name him phonetically is probably inherently an outcast, due to the hearse they drive him to school in, the fact that his parents are first cousins and the 3-wheeled trailer that they all live in — so they could have named him "Kick Me" and it wouldn't have made much of a difference.

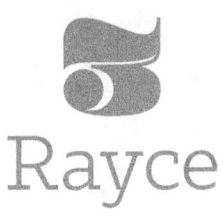

# Rayce

I'm not going to say, "Now I've seen it all," because this journey has just begun, and I have a feeling that you and I will see far more ridiculous shit together, but naming your kid a verb?!? Jesus Christ…

At least I assume it's pronounced "race." You never know with inbreds and their concocted names. I suppose it could be "racy." Maybe the kid came out in a purple teddy and a come-hither smile on his face. Or her face, since we have no fucking idea what gender this child is.

More than likely, though, his parents are NASCAR fans. In other words, he will never have a job that pays taxes. The other miniature rednecks at his babysitter's trailer will probably think his name is cool, and so as long as he stays in the South he may get out of this thing alive. But God help him if Momma runs off with a yankee and he has to move north of the Mason-Dixon line.

Here's a tip for you potential parents that plan on naming your kid something stupid — misspelling and/or adding letters to a common verb does not a name make. Much like Rayce, the words Juymp, Ruun, Fyte and Fliye are not names either. They're spelling errors.

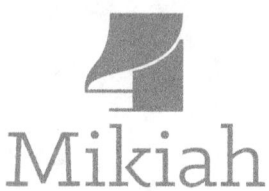

# Mikiah

This name is pronounced "ma-ki-uh" according to the dipshits that made it up and saddled an innocent child with it. I Googled it to see if it had any meaning. Then I realized that doing so made me nearly as stupid as the parents, since I knew damn well before typing it in that no one has any idea what the fuck it meant, because it was fabricated. I might as well have looked up the word "farzenquietzelish."

My question for these parents, as with all of the parents that make up words to name their kids, is why? There are millions of names already in existence that don't sound like the scientific name for a large, colorful bird — why not choose one of those?

Is it because you want your kid to be "different?" Don't worry — she will be. No matter what you name her, she will be the only one at school with parents who always have to wear helmets and who shit their pants while watching her "Math Counts" competitions.

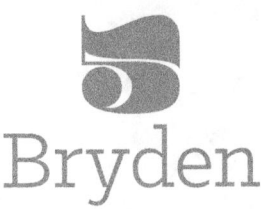

# Bryden

This is exactly the type of name that led to the creation of this book. A perfect example of a ridiculous woman and her spineless husband going way over the line. You and I both know that this was her idea, and he was too pussy whipped to tell her the truth — that this name is complete bullshit and no one should ever have to endure a life with this name.

These made up names are the worst of them all — so much worse than overused names like Kaitlynn or McKenzie. At least those names were cute at one time — before every 3rd couple decided to use them.

**Side note:** *If you are thinking of naming your daughter Kaitlynn or McKenzie, you should know that she will take the cock on film some day. Proven fact.*

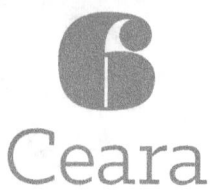

# Ceara

*I don't even know how to begin forming my mouth to pronounce this word jumble. See-ra? Sierra? Shay-ra? See-are-a? Does it make a 'ch' sound, like 'ciao?' Is it a fucking acronym? A palindrome? Aren't there too many vowels? WHAT THE FUCK!?!*

That is exactly what I would say if I were a teacher doing roll call on the first day of school and this pile of shit crept up. Then I would send it to the corner and make it think about what its parents have done.

Let's assume that this is pronounced "Sierra." That would make the most sense on its face (which is most likely why it's NOT actually pronounced this way). Why not just name her "Sierra?" Do they think there will be an overabundance of those in her school? How many of them do YOU know? Why spell it all funky and confuse the rest of us trying to read it?

I'll tell you why — because people who do this shit have never done a god damned thing in their lives that will leave a mark on this world, so they think that they will get the attention they crave by trying to make their kid unique.

Either that, or they're just assholes. Trust me. I know my own kind.

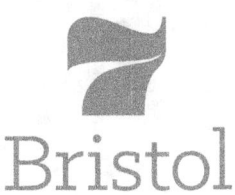

# Bristol

As you know, this is the name of one Sarah Palin's daughters. Because of that, it may soon be as common — and annoying — as McKenzie, amongst the already fucked up & annoying conservative right.

I read that they actually named her after Bristol Bay, "where the family fishes." I shit you not. I fish at Turkey Holler, but I don't go naming my fucking kid Turkey, now do I? No, I don't. I guess it's a good thing they aren't ocean anglers, otherwise we might have a Gulf Palin or a Pacific Palin.

And that's not even the half of it — her other kids are Trig, Track, Willow and Piper. Jesus...she and her snow blower husband have single handedly fucked up 5 entire human beings with the stroke of a pen on a birth certificate. Not only did she go and name all of her kids after random places she's been and words that confuse her, she also went and made herself famous. Now she has opened the floodgates for the entire world to heckle the little bastards, and not just the other kids at Moose Knuckle Elementary. It's almost as if she's trying to ruin their lives.

Sarah Palin is definitely the first, and possibly forever the most prolific, inductee into the "My Poorly Named Kids Never Had A Fighting Chance Hall Of Fame." Since she had about as good a shot of being president as John Hinckley, I guess it's not so bad. At least she made it to the top of the heap in some arena. I wonder if she can see Russia from up there?

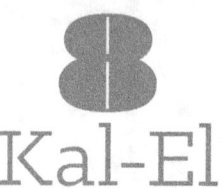

# Kal-El

Fuck you for this, Nicolas Cage! Fuck you straight to Hell!

For those of you who aren't 37-year-old virgins who ejaculate directly onto a spread of open comic books on your futon, Kal-El is the birth name of Superman. Back when he was just Superboy, but I guess his teachers weren't down with calling him Superboy.

Maybe Kal-El was the name of the lake where his parents fished. I don't fucking know. I had to look that shit up on Wikipedia to even tell you about Superboy.

This one really hits home because I have a cousin who named his kid Kal-El. He lives in his car and has been looking for work for around two years. My cousin, not the kid. Not yet, anyway.

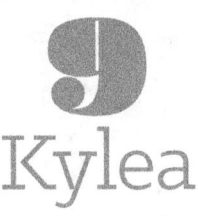

# Kylea

It's going to get to the point with some of these names that you people are going to call bullshit. You are going to say that there is no way that I actually stumbled upon the name in question, and that I made it up just to fill a book. Not true, although I don't blame you a bit for your skepticism.

You might envision a beautiful woman with a flower in her hair in the islands when you see the name Kylea, as I'm sure her mother did. I, on the other hand, imagine something like this:

"Kylea. KYLEA! Go get Tanner and Skylar and get in the God dayum truck! I swear to God if you don't stop running around this store and get to the truck I am going whup all your asses! No! NO, you caint have no cigarette lighters — you ain't even old enough to smoke yet. Now get your asses to the TRUCK!"

Poor Kylea. Momma thought her name was "real purdy." Guess what, Momma? It's not. It sounds like some shit you made up to top Becky's daughter's name (Machara) because she was born 6 months before Kylea and everyone was telling her how cute her baby's name was. Right? Fuck Becky, huh?

Bitch don't even have no
man to take care of her.

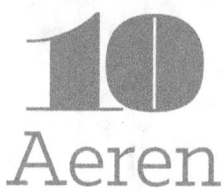

# Aeren

Can you guess how Mommy and Daddy pronounce this gem? No? Just like Erin. Don't you want to grab them both by their skinny little throats and scream,

> *Why don't you just name*
> *the fucking kid erin then?!?!*

Of course you do. If you know the parents of an Aeren, I encourage you to do just that.

The "unique spelling of a normal name" syndrome pisses me off more than anything else. I it worse than total name fabrication, because the work is already done for these assholes, then they go and fuck it all up. Basically, it's a big April Fool's prank to the rest of a society, EVERY SINGLE TIME someone has to write down her name. "Oops! Fooled ya! I scrambled up all the letters on ya. HAHAHA! This makes my kid unique!!"

It really doesn't. It just makes you a contemptible asshole.

# 11
## Taeron

If I am not mistaken, this is the capital of Iran. Wait — no? Oh, it's actually an American kid's name? Shit...

I wonder how you actually do pronounce this one. Tay-ron? Tie-ron? Tie-rone? Tie-ee-ron? Tuh-ron? Tire Iron? Or maybe it is something else altogether. I vote for the latter. Nothing is apparently out of bounds for the anyone who gave their kid this name. It's probably pronounced "Tron."

I have no idea if this is a feminine or masculine name. I read it somewhere, and the context clues did nothing to clear it up. It was something like "Taeron seen a ghost and runned away." As a rational person, I am assuming it's a male, but obviously we are not dealing with rational people here, so who knows.

What I do know is that it is not only a burden on this kid, it is a waste of my fucking time (yours too!) to name a kid shit like this. It'll take forever for the nurse at the doctor's office to snarl out every pronunciation, and the dumb shit will most likely not respond until she gets it exactly right — as if there's some other fucktard with a similar name out there. We'll all suffer in the end.

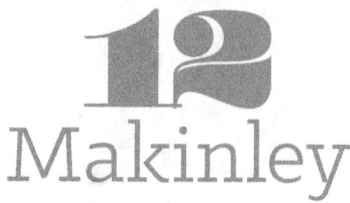

# Makinley

McKinley is an awful name for a little girl. Makinley is a God damned travesty.

You see, McKinley was probably pretty cute the first 7 to 8 thousand times it was done. Now, it's just like McKenzie, Kaitlyn and Emma — WAY too fucking common.

So what's the remedy when you just HAVE to name your little princess McKinley, because you have been planning on naming your little girl that since you were playing dollies in the sandbox? Fuck the spelling up, of course! That creates a whole new name that only YOUR little darling has. She's all cute and extraordinary and unique! What a special girl Makinley is!

Yeah — because that's what you want — an 8 year old that's different from all of the other kids. As if that's not a breeding ground for childhood terrorism.

Plus, not for nothing, it's really close to Makin' Love, which is not what you want to think about when there's an 8-year-old girl involved.

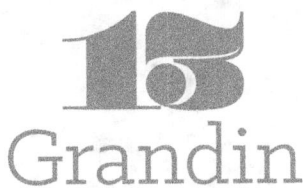

# 15

# Grandin

Want to ensure your kid's name is a piece of dick? Pick it out of a parenting magazine. Christ, talk about the cesspools of the naming world. Some misguided freelance twat making 5 cents a word churned out a naming article that included this gem. God help this poor girl.

I'm guessing the name came from Temple Grandin, a quasi-famous writer, professor and autism activist. If you have ever fucking heard of Temple Grandin, it's probably because HBO made a movie about her with Claire Danes in it. If, despite HBO and Claire's best efforts, you still haven't heard of her, well, join the fucking club. Neither has most of the rest of the world.

Temple Grandin is by all accounts a really swell gal. Superfuckingduper. But you dickhead parents realize that Grandin was her LAST name, right? Temple Grandin's own fucking parents didn't even name HER Grandin — they named her Temple.

Your little shit of a daughter isn't a Grandin and very likely will never resemble Temple Grandin in any way at all, just like naming my daughter Ruth or Aaron (of, if she's like you fucksticks, "Aeren") wouldn't make her any better at hitting home runs.

And did you ever think that the CHILD HERSELF may not, I don't know, WANT to be associated with Temple Grandin any more than, say, Warren G. Harding or Martin Luther King or Billie Jean Fucking King or Ryan Seacrest or whoever the fuck you want your daughter to remind you of since apparently just being herself is not enough for you?

News flash: kids aren't fucking pets or automobiles or anything else we decide to give stupid, whimsical, aren't-I-just-so-clever names to. They're actual humans with feelings and peers and identities and all that shit. STOP NAMING YOUR CHILDREN AS IF THEY'RE A FUCKING PIECE OF PROPERTY.

Plus, "Grandin" sounds like an angry German taking a shit. This is the worst name I have seen to date.

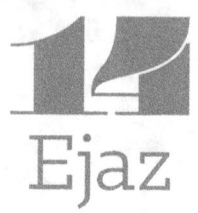

# Ejaz

Well, that didn't last very long.
THIS is now the worst name
I have seen to date.

I don't even know where to begin with this one. This sounds more like an expression of shock than a name. Where does a shitty parent even come up with something like this? Do they love electronic jazz music? Did they name him after the load that Daddy shot in Mommy's womb? Are they addicted to heroin?

The problem is that these parents think they're so fucking cute when they do shit like this. I guarantee you they both giggled and high-fived each other when they came up with it. They tell everyone within earshot his name, because they are so fucking proud that they made it up and he is the only one in the world with this name. I bet they are more proud of the name than they are of the fucking kid himself.

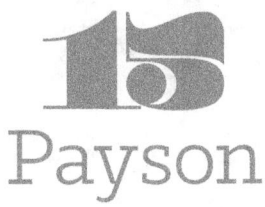

# Payson

I don't know how I actually finished writing this book. I have blood pressure issues, and I get angrier and closer to a stroke with every entry. When I read about fucking Payson here, for example, the entire left side of my face went numb and I shit my pants.

These fuckers seemingly just removed a letter and replaced it with a different letter — so Payton becomes Payson. Fucking clever, huh?

Most of you less observant folk would not realize that what we have here is called a "compromise." You see, I read this name in a magazine, and the magazine said that little Payson here lives in Indiana. Obviously Daddy's favorite football team is the Colts and therefore his favorite player is Payton Manning, Manning having previously been the long time leader of the Colts. Mommy was not willing to give in to naming him after a famous football player (and rightfully so), but in an equally ridiculous move, wanted to name him "something unique" (now I hate her even worse than Dad….100 times worse).

I don't know exactly what happened in the following minutes, hours, days and weeks, but somehow both of their brains became entangled and they Frankensteined together this piece of shit name.

I hope little Payson grows up to hate sports, hate other kids, hate uniqueness and most of all, hate his parents.

# 16
# Boston

Yep — a whole new avenue has apparently opened up with kid names — naming them after your favorite city, sports team and/or 70s rock band. This fucking kid hit the trifecta!

I am willing to accept that certain city names could work as kid names (although none come to mind), but Boston is not one of them. Unless, of course, your child comes into the world as a boorish, crass, old man. Then Boston would be perfect.

I am going to go out on a limb and say that this kid was named after the Red Sox or the Celtics (WICKED AWESOME!) namely because he was born long before the tragic bombings at the Boston Marathon (and no, that's still not a good fucking reason to name your kid Boston). It makes sense, as fans of those 2 teams are perennially out of touch with reality when it comes to the "importance" of sports, and would not hesitate to see their child as yet another sports collectible rather than a living, breathing, miniature human being.

The good news is, Boston will have company when he gets older, as the decaying assembly-line plant he works the graveyard shift at his entire life will probably have a few Bostons, a couple of Bradys, one Celtic and a guy named Fuck New York.

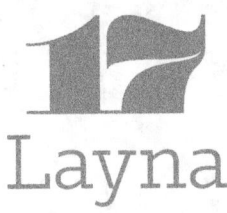

# Layna

Ever notice how most of these cutesy little bullshit names that these awful parents come up with these days ends with the "uh" sound? Layna, Kirrah, Soraya, Kylea, Ceara, etc. How ironic is it that these assholes are trying to be "unique", but instead their kid's name sounds like all of the rest of the parents that are trying the same shit? Should have gone with Ann, assholes.

So I saw this name, and I had never heard it before, so I Googled it and what I found proves my fucking point EXACTLY! The following is an entry from the Urban Dictionary:

*Layna* — *A beautiful, funny, loving, hott, sexy, crazy, party naked kind of girl whose best friend is almost always lesbian/Bi, usually with red or brown hair.*

See? Your daughter is already a slut. She will spend her entire life living up to others' expectations, and those expectations are that she be an alcoholic party girl who is sensational at fellatio. She can do nothing to avoid it, and it's all your fault. I hope you're happy.

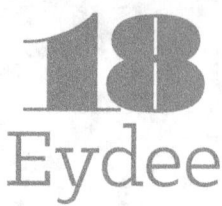

# Eydee

Another dandy from a parenting magazine. It seems to me that no matter how cute your little bundle of joy is, if he or she does not have some fucked up moniker, the kid isn't getting in the magazine. And we all know that the parents that name their kids stupid shit like this are the same kind that crave the attention of having their little doll in a big time magazine. Even though the magazine is so shitty that you can get a two-year subscription for like $11.50.

This has to be one of the worst I have ever seen. I cannot begin to imagine what they were thinking when they invented this name. Seriously — no jokes or spin on this one. I can't find a way to make my mind go to whatever places theirs went to when this seemed like a word that should become a child's name. Sorry, I don't have that part in my brain.

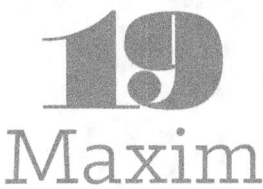

# Maxim

The creation of this name was probably in the exact same mold as the creation of all of these others — vanity — but I like to believe that Mommy insisted on something unique, and when Daddy threw this out there as a joke she bit hook, line and sinker. She had no idea that Daddy came up with it while reading a softcore titty magazine of the same name while he was taking a shit 5 minutes earlier.

This is not the most awful thing to name your son, but it makes the book due to the fact that it is also the name of the world's biggest "lad mag," where douchebags of all ages learn new ways to drink beer, pull tail, buy clothes they can't afford and basically grow into even bigger douchebags. Even if that wasn't the impetus of how he got the name, it had to at least come into the discussion. And when it did, even Mommy ignored the fact that her son may as well be named GQ, Details or Stuff.

I like the name Max just fine, and I am fairly certain that this is what he will be called 99% of the time. But if the other kids get a whiff of his real name, he may have to pay his dues a little bit. The good news is that a kid whose father had the rocks to name him after a smut rag is probably so full of inherited testosterone that he could kick the shit out of any and all comers.

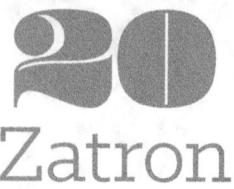

# Zatron

Obviously we are all thinking the same thing, right? And to answer your question, yes...Zatron is a robot. Well, not technically, but I bet he has to have robotic emotions to deal with the constant barrage of teasing and name calling he has been forced to endure.

This was a kid that I actually met myself. Here's a shocker — I met him while working with troubled youths. He was in the behavioral disorder classroom. I assume it was because he was constantly having to swing on fools for making fun of his name.

I don't know what ever became of little Zatron. I would bet dollars to donuts that he is serving hard time right about now. And if so, many people will blame it on society or growing up in a bad environment. I blame it on his mother. All of it.

If he's Michael, he doesn't have to kick ass to survive. Michael is a businessman. Zatron is a felon.

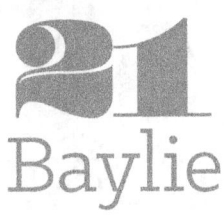

# Baylie

I am writing a letter to my congressman as soon as I am done here, asking him to submit a bill that decriminalizes the aggravated assault upon anyone doing shit like this to their innocent child. You should be able to beat people up for giving their children stupid names.

Jesus, people — she's just a little girl. She never did anything to anyone. What did she do to you to deserve this? Are you bitter about the labor pains? Is she an accident that you are trying to "get back" at? Do you just hate children in general?

Nah — we all know the truth is that you're just too fucking common and you're trying to make sure that your kid doesn't end up a nobody like you did. It's just like the Dad that wants to play sports vicariously through his boys because he was a turd on the field himself.

**Guess what? You made her stand out all right — which is exactly the kind of thing that could make her be:**

**(A)** A sorority slut that inhales jock-boner regularly

**(B)** A goth freak that goes by her middle name, which is probably Rayven or Starrr

**(C)** A juvenile delinquent and an adult loser that hates your guts for painting a target on her.

Baylie is a brand of delicious booze (spelled incorrectly), not a child's name. Don't name your kid after booze, no matter how much of it you drank while you were pregnant.

# Nevaeh

I'm gonna get letters about this one for sure, but God dammit - someone has to stand up against this shit!

Bet you can't guess where they came up with this name. Look closely. Think hard. Got it yet? No, of course you don't, because no one would ever think to spell a baby's fucking name backward in order to figure out the meaning behind it. Yeah, that's right — it's Heaven spelled backward. Jesus Christ.

Where can parents possibly go from here? (Other than the local strip club to pick up Nevaeh after her shift ends because her 1992 Nissan Sentra won't start again, and she doesn't want to have to blow another bouncer to get home like she did last week.) They've made up words, given regular names extra letters, removed letters from regular names and replaced them with different ones, named their kids after cities or sports teams and now this shit — normally awful names made even more awful by spelling them backward.

I have never seen anyone go so far out of their way to screw something up. Ever. I can't even fathom a way that anyone could take a more fucked up route to get to a child's name. That being said, it's gotten fairly common. Maybe the world is, in fact, coming to an end.

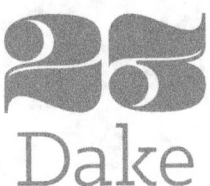

# Dake

This is not a name, no matter how you slice it. It's just not.

At best it's the non-name Drake, broken down into more of a non-name than it already was. At worst, it's word pulled directly from Jabberwocky.

No matter what, it's a symbol of 2 people's undying stupidity and their attempted destruction of an innocent child.

I am basically at a loss for words. This would be atrocious as a *middle* name, which is the name usually reserved for the "family heirloom" name or the "crazy idea" name. As a first name, it's nothing short of criminal.

It sounds like food. Like something you'd put on a salad.

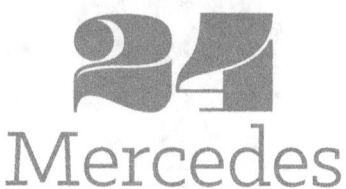

# Mercedes

I included this name out of necessity, more than shock. We've all probably met someone named Mercedes — it's not all that uncommon anymore. But it would be like ignoring the elephant in the room not to call out the people naming their kids after expensive cars and fancy brand names.

The following are not only NOT names, they are also things that people who name their kids after them will NEVER be able to afford (Note: the following list is NOT all-inclusive. If one of these things triggers a thought of another item in a similar category, it's not to be used as a human's name either.):

Mercedes, Lexus, Chanel, Gucci, Guess, Fendi, Porsche (or any spelling thereof), Bentley, Aston, Avalon, Louis Vuitton, Rolex, Cartier, Tag Heuer, Hilfiger, Ralph Lauren (although separately each name is fine for a boy and girl, respectively), Hermes, Saks, Prada, Hennessey, Cristal, Dom, Vera Wang, and/or Armani.

And just so we're clear, the following items, although you may be able to afford them, are not baby names either (again, not an all-inclusive list — use good judgment):

Ford, Chevy, Toyota, Mercury, Chrysler, Sears, American Eagle (unless you're Native American — then you have the green light), Mossimo, Panama Jack, Old Navy, Sam's Choice, Old Spice, Brut, Old Crow, Ten High and/or Pabst.

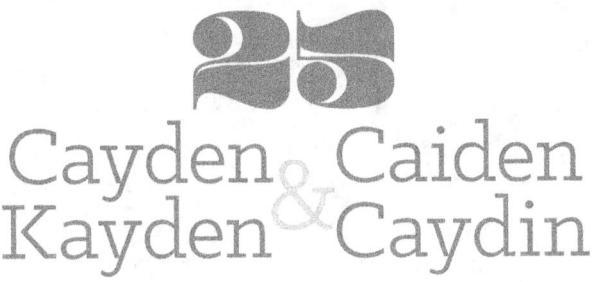

# Cayden Caiden
# Kayden & Caydin

...and tons of other fucked up spellings that this one can be found under.

This "one-sex-fits-all" pseudonym is popping up fairly often these days. It must have been on a soap opera, reality show, in People magazine or on Perez Hilton's shitty blog. Those are the places where people that name their kids shit like this spend all of their free time.

On a whim I searched for the meaning of this name. Turns out it's a mash-up of a couple of Irish names, and it means "battle." Let's hope you are what you're named in this case, because the little fuckers that get this one pinned on them are in for a lifetime of battles.

Here's to you little Cadens of the world. Mom and Dad fucked you up from the get go — let's hope you're strong enough to "battle" your way out of it.

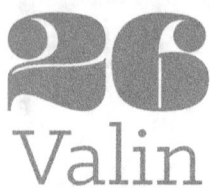

# Valin

Ho-ly shit. Fucking Valin. I have to assume that this is some character from Star Wars, Star Trek or The Matrix. Please, someone tell me that's the case and the parents didn't just pull this out of thin air?

Not that it would necessarily be any better if it were from a movie. Naming your kid after a Klingon is equally sinful to naming him or her like these people probably did — by eating a bowl of Alphabet soup, taking a shit and randomly putting together the floating letters in the toilet that survived your stomach acid.

As I often do, I looked this one up to see what the meaning behind it could have been. Believe it or not, I actually found one — and it's pure fucking gold. You see, Mommy and Daddy, you named your son something that you thought was bold and original, but it turns out that Valin means "Monkey King" in Hindu.

## Monkey. Fucking. King.

I bet you $100 this is news to these parents. No way someone knows that shit and still names their kid Valin. So...SURPRISE! Hope you can swallow that lump in your throat, pretend you knew it all along and somehow keep a straight face when you tell everyone that it's really honorable in India to be the king of the apes.

Hey Valin, do us all a favor, will ya? Take a shit in your claw and fling it at your folks. They deserve it.

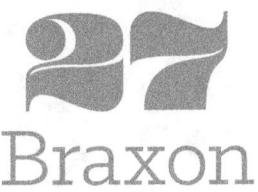

# Braxon

After a while, it seems like these all sound alike. For each new name I include, I actually have to go back and look to see if I have previously lambasted the parents. That's how fucking stupid these names are — the parents' goal is to make little precious different and special by throwing a created name on him. Instead, he now sounds like most of the others, and Michael and David are the unique ones.

Braxon is shit. Any time you come to an "X" in a name, you know the name is probably a pathetic quasi-creative concoction by a mom and dad who love nothing more than the smell of their own farts. In fact, most names containing the letter "X" are created just to be different. True story.

**I am guessing that this name came from one of two things:**

**(A)** Braxon Industries is the name of the factory that Daddy works in

**(B)** Mom and Dad took a birthing class, heard about Braxton-Hicks contractions, thought that sounded cool, fucked up the spelling and...voila!

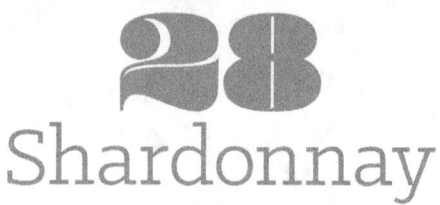

# Shardonnay

I'm not a wine drinker myself. Gave it up years ago, plus, as this book has already shown you, I'm not classy enough to be an oenophile. Yeah, motherfuckers, I said "oenophile." That means wine-lover.

And you know what? I also SPELLED IT FUCKING CORRECTLY, because even a whiskey-swilling dipshit like me knows that nothing takes away the aura of sophistication that you thought you were giving your child naming her after fine wine than FUCKING MISSPELLING IT.

I know, I know. You didn't actually misspell it, right? You just chose a unique, personal spelling. Because a girl with a misspelled alcoholic beverage for her name signals "special" to the world.

Do you know where your daughter is right now? Because I do. She's sucking cock in the VIP room of a strip club. That's what she's doing, and she's doing it solely because you named her Shardonnay.

I might be wrong if she's under like 12 years old still, but even if that's the case, watch her in the passenger's seat as you drive by the nearest strip club. She's already staring too long at the sign, fucking longing, feeling the pull of her future profession. And it's all because you named her Shardonnay, you fucking dickhead.

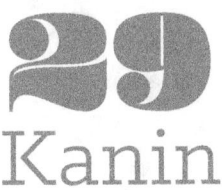

# Kanin

Well, this certainly is an original name, huh? Nothing like naming your kid after a Civil War era death-weapon! Yay Mom and Dad!

Or should I just say yay Dad, as this has a man's insistence and a woman's spelling written all over it. Dad heard the names Gunnar and Hunter (probably while his buddies were talking about their kids) and wanted to come up with something even more original, but cooler and sounding even more like a true man's man. The result — Cannon. Mom agreed only if she could spell it her way. You know, to sell it to her Mom's group. I bet they think it's, "Soooo adorable!"

OR, it's pronounced KAY-nin, in which case, of course, his classmates are already calling him Gay-nin. Outstanding.

Actually this name is so stupid and not name-like, that I have no idea it's really a boy's name — I am just guessing on that one. I sure hope it is. As much shit as a boy will get for this name, it's not survivable by a little girl.

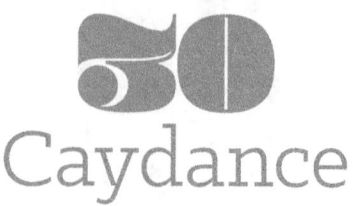

# Caydance

This is one that has been popping up WAY too frequently lately. It's also even more annoying than most, because it has hundreds of different spellings — Kadence, Kaydence, Caidence, Kaidance, Kaedinz — all for the same fucking pronunciation.

I have no idea how this one grew in popularity. I would think that only military families and marching band nerds would name their kids shit like this. Why would anyone else want to name their daughter something that means "rhythmic" and is only used when discussing some sort of marching or yelling?

You know what? I give up. In fact, I hope you dipshits start naming your kids after military terms more often. I hope I start seeing kids named Ambush, Infiltration, Siege and Bayonet.

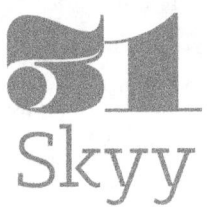

## Skyy

Earthh. Waterr. Windd.
Heavenn. Cloudd. Rainn.

See? Those all sound like shit too — no matter how many times you repeat the last letter.

Oh wait, but then it wouldn't be spelled just like the mid-grade vodka you drank a gallon of the night you got pregnant with this precious little accident.

You are a whore and an alcoholic.

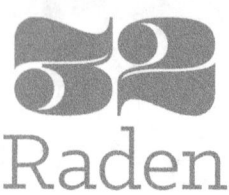

# Raden

Totally fucking made up. I mean — this one is not even CLOSE to a real name. Hell, it's not even close to a real word!

The closest word, in my mind, would be "raven." That would have been shitty enough as a name, but these idiots even topped that. Maybe it was just a clerical error on the birth certificate and they were too fucking lazy to cut the red tape to change it. Nah...fuck that. I'm not letting them off the hook. They took a verbal shit and smeared it on their kid.

This is another one that I can't figure out — whether it's a boy's or girl's name. A boy would certainly get his ass kicked 365 days per year — 366 on a leap year — so I hope it's a girl's name. It would suck for her too, but she would be less likely to end up in a wheelchair because of it.

Hey, everybody. Word to the wise here. "Aidan" is a real name. Making up a name that rhymes with "Aidan" by sticking a random consonant on the front of it — Jayden, Raden, Cayden, Fadin', Hatin', Baitin', Participatin', Conversay-in' — that makes you not only a prick, but an unoriginal prick too.

When your children grow up, they will hate you. Unless they change their name, in which case they'll only hate you when they think about their childhood.

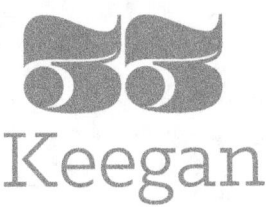

# Keegan

I've seen a lot of these traditional Irish names lately — Keegan, Teagan, Seamus, etc. Just because you're a shit-your-pants drunk doesn't mean you're REALLY Irish, so quit naming your kids Irish names.

And while we're on the subject, all of you cutesy parents that are naming your daughters McKenzie, Makenzie, McKinley and shit like that — "Mac" is of Irish descent and means "son of." Unless you are pretty sure that your little girl is gonna have a pecker added later in life, don't name her Mac-anything.

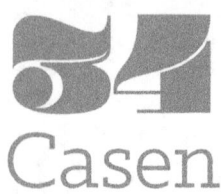

# Casen

## And the hits keep comin'...

I don't believe that parents who do this type of thing even think for a second to put themselves in the shoes of the kid at age, say...11. Can you imagine being an 11 year old boy and having a dainty little piece-of-shit name like Casen? If you can't, let me paint you a picture — Casen will be getting teased and pummelled by Michael, David and Josh.

I searched for the origin of this one, and it wasn't just made up out of thin air. Worse, almost — it's Scandinavian. Not that Scandinavian is inherently bad, but I am betting that Mom and Pop have no idea what or where Scandinavia is. They probably think it's the name of someplace in Lord-of-the-Rings world. Plus, Ikea furniture is cheap and shitty and you know it is.

If you're American, stick to the classics, people. If you want to get creative, go back to a 50s name book and pick one of those. Ernest is fine. Ingmar is not.

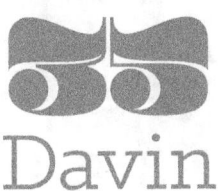

# Davin

Remember that president we had with the first name Davin? Or that CEO of that Fortune 500 company named Davin? No? Of course you didn't. That's because you don't hear about any kids named Davin growing up & excelling at shit, do you?

Why? Because Davin is a last name, not a first name — unless you think you're super clever like the parents of this kid I read about here. Sheesh — Pretty soon we are going to be talking about kids named Schmidt, Johnson and McDonald.

Actually, who am I kidding? I'm one THOUSAND percent certain that's already happening. That's why this book is merely the first of many, many volumes you'll be reading.

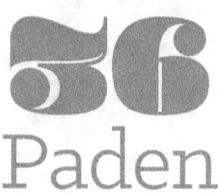

# Paden

Wow. This one is not only Irish, it's an Irish LAST name. So...these people doubled up on the bullshit. Excellent work. Your kid's name is not only the worst in his school, it's one of the most fucked up names in all of America!

Who knows — maybe instead these assholes are in the category of people naming their kids after towns, as there is a Paden, Oklahoma and a Paden, Mississippi. The combined population of both towns is 552 — so if they did name him after one of them, shit just got infinitely worse. Most likely, it's another Payton Manning fan or one of those Aidan-rhymers. Or both.

I never went to school with any kids with names as shitty as Paden. If I had, I promise you his life would have been a living hell. I would have made it so, personally. Is that wrong? Absolutely — but welcome to the real world, Mom and Dad. Kids are brutal. Even more so to other kids with stupid names.

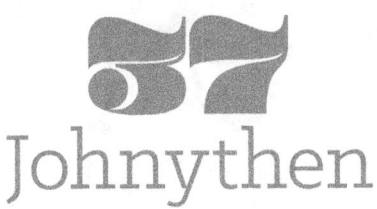

# Johnythen

What is there to say about a alphabetical debacle like this? God damn — this has to be the single worst butchering of a classic name that I've ever seen.

The people that did this are possibly worst type of all. I hate people that name their kids off the wall, shitty names, but I do have to give them a sliver of credit for being ballsy (and don't get me wrong — that credit is far outweighed by the damage it will do to the kid). People like Johnythen's parents here want to go "out on a limb," but can't quite work up the gumption to do so — so they give their kid a name that sounds like a traditional name, but is spelled like a bag full of dicks.

> Johnythen will be fine as long as no one ever SEES his name. If they do…he's in for a rough ride.

Johnny-thin sounds like a drug that keeps you awake for days while you suck dicks for money in a truck-stop bathroom to get the money to pay your drug dealer for more drugs.

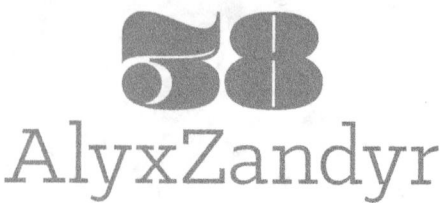

# AlyxZandyr

Unreal. Take everything I just said about Johnython, multiply it by 5,000, and apply it to this abortion. It took me seven different retypes to get this one correct.

I am considering legal action as a concerned citizen. There is little chance of this child's survival without intervention by someone who cares. His parents obviously don't.

Sometimes I think of what would be a true and realistic punishment for parents who name their kids something like this. I mean, all joking aside, terrible as it is, you can't kill them or even strip the kid away and put him in foster care for this. Unfortunately.

I've come up with this: Once every 90 days, the father and mother should both be shot in the middle of the back with one of those crowd-control bean bag guns. That, or a Taser blast every 60 days. I think that's enough punishment to let them continue living their lives as normal, but also to be in some constant, if mild, physical ache as penance.

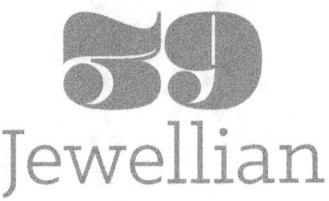

# Jewellian

I must admit before I start bashing this one that I hate the name Jillian. Not sure why — it's a completely irrational hatred, but I have always hated it just the same.

I have also always hated the name Jewel. I DO know why I hate this one — because it's a fucking rock and/or a shitty singer, not a name.

Then I come across this hybrid, fucked-up loanblend that has been stuck on some poor child for her to battle with for the rest of her life. Lots of people will call her Jillian out of pure confusion. Others will call her Jewel-lyin or Jew-well-ian. Or, of course, Julian. Most will likely fall to the floor clutching their chests and gasping for air as they try to contort their tongues to pronounce it.

No one — and I mean NO ONE — wins when you invent a name like this for your kid. Except us. Then we get to write books about how shitty you are.

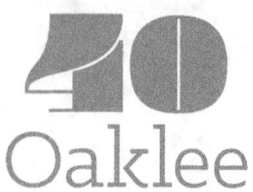

# Oaklee

Reminder — I didn't make any of this shit up.

I think I saw the name "Oakley" once, but that could have been on a pair of sunglasses where it belonged. Oaklee, on the other hand? Not sure this sort of tragedy has ever occurred before.

I would have bet $100 that this was a name these people invented for a boy. Turns out, I would have been wrong. Of course, people that do shit like this are about as predictable as Kim Jong Un on angel dust. Oaklee is, in fact, a poor little girl.

I am positive that Mom was inundated with compliments of how "beautiful" this name is. Guess what, Mom? Your friends are all liars. They don't believe this — but what else can you say to someone who drops a bomb on you like, "This is my little baby girl. Her name is Oaklee!"

I'll tell you what else you can say. You can say,

> *Fuck you. Fuck you for naming your poor little child such a shitty thing.*
> *I hope you rot in the deepest part of Hell.*

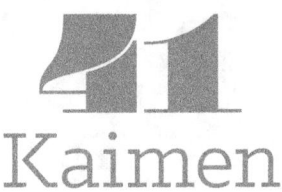

# Kaimen

To the untrained eye, this is merely another invented and misspelled piece of shit name. But of all of the names that I've written about so far, this one sent up the quickest red flag for something NOT to name your child. Why? Read on...

The most important thing to think about (that couples never do) when trying to name your kid something "unique," is, "How will the other kids use this concoction to make fun of my child?" Try these childhood killers on for size:

Kaimen her face, Kaimen her mouth, Kamien her hair, Kamien his ass and left him lying on the prison cell shaking and sobbing — get the picture yet? This name is a fucking nightmare for any child, boy or girl. Sorry, mom — no one's going to be envisioning the Cayman Islands. They're going to be envisioning hot, viscous semen, ejaculated inside your children. Way to fucking go.

Of course Mom and Dad will jump up and down and shout. "That's not how you pronounce it! It's pronounced Kie-man!!"

Yeah. Whatever. Tell that to the 11 year old taunting your kid for the 100th consecutive day — I'm sure he'll realize the errors of his mispronunciations and stop.

And for the cherry on top, I Googled this and it popped up in the Urban Dictionary. The definition is as follows:

***Kaimen:*** *a saucy piece of meat that every imagineable form of life wants to get their hands on. Example: "Wow. Did you see that Kaimen over there? I'd fuck that!"*

Need I say more?

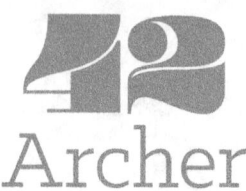

# Archer

Unless your kid is born with a bow and arrow in his hands, this name is beyond ridiculous. I am assuming the parents have some sort of connection to archery. Maybe they competed in the Olympics. Maybe his Dad was Cupid. It doesn't fucking matter — it's a stupid idea for a name.

You should never name a kid after shit you like to do or how you make your living. It's just plain stupid. If everyone did this, we would have kids running around named Construction, Baller, Sheetrocker, Attorney, Roofer and Rapist.

Of course, odds are we already do, I just haven't stumbled on them yet.

**Side note:** *If the child is named after Sterling Archer, the alcoholic nymphomaniac secret agent that is the namesake of the Archer show on FX, then disregard the above, as this is totally acceptable and even encouraged.*

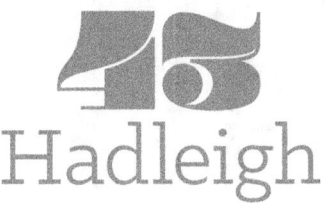

# Hadleigh

This name was actually posted on a baby names forum, with the headline, "Would she get laughed at for these names?" The other names this woman listed were Sonnet and Delaney.

The answer is yes - of course she will. In fact, you damn well knew it before you asked, or the question wouldn't have entered your mind. You never see anyone ask if their kid will get laughed at for the name Ann or Stacey, right? Because you say them out loud and they don't sound like shit other than names (like types of poems or the sound of a frat boy vomiting out the window of his Jeep).

You just want at least one person to tell you, "No. No, those are BEAUTIFUL names!" Then you have all of the confirmation your tiny little self-centered brain needs to justify this bullshit. Because you're a sad fucking person.

Not surprisingly this woman did not write back other than to say "thanks for your opinions, I am leaning toward Sonnet." Well, I'll tell you right here, ma'am — that is a fucking stupid name too, and your daughter will suffer in some way or another every day of her life that she has to interact with a new person.

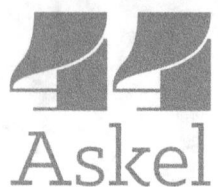

# Askel

## I shit you not.

This is the most unattractive name that I have ever heard. Ever. The only thing that it has going for it is that it is apparently attached to a boy and not a girl. Hey...that's something, right? No. No, it's not.

What do you think the mean little boys at Askel's school are gonna come up with for a nickname? My bet is Askel the Asshole. But kids today are pretty clever and more sinister than I ever was — it may be something much more brutal.

I hope more than anything in the world that little Askel has a halfway decent middle name to go by when he is old enough to shun his parents and make his own decisions. More than likely, however, his middle name is something like Borscht, Carburetor, Haagenfrudel or Cunt.

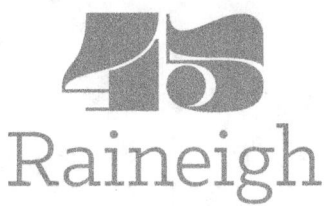

# Raineigh

Some names are made up with good intentions, despite the fact that they are truly horrible and will be a huge burden on their children.

Other names, like Raineigh here (pronounced "Rainy") are nothing more than fucked up people going out of their way to come up with the most fucked up shit they can think of. I hope at one point in her life, a nurse or teacher or whatever reads the child's name, stops, looks up from the paper, stares straight at the parent and says, "Really? Why. Fucking why. Why did you do this? Do you feel smart and clever? Because you're not. You're just a selfish asshole."

I am guessing the mother that did this to her daughter is either a hippe-wanna-be or a Wiccan. Either way, she's an awful, awful person. Not for her lifestyle, but for her dragging her kid into it before she's old enough to make the decision for herself.

Raineigh is a forecast, not a name. And a shitty forecast at that. There's nothing good that can come out of naming your kid Raineigh.

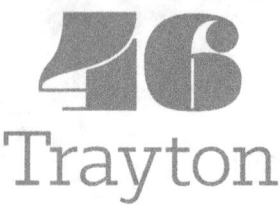

# Trayton

If you are going to name your kid something weird and made up, at least try to make it a little difficult for another kid to make fun of it. Or, if you decide to name your kid Trayton, at least make damn sure he's never one ounce overweight or he will be called Two Ton Trayton for the rest of his life.

Besides the ripe possibility of damaging nicknames, this is just a flat out ridiculous name. I looked it up — something the parents apparently never did — and guess what it means? A settlement near trees. Pretty, huh? And not even in some fucked up language like Swahili or Farsi — it's an English expression.

A little research goes a long way, people. You thought you were cute, but you ended up naming your kid after a group of hovels in the woods. Nice going.

Trayton sounds like the name of a robot. A robot with shitty parents.

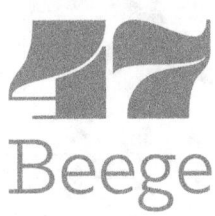

# Beege

Where do you even begin with a disaster like this? Is it pronounced like the fantastic 70s group? Or is it "Beej"? Or maybe even like B.J. (don't put anything past assholes that do shit like this).

Congrats, Mom and Dad. You wanted something unique. I am willing to bet that Beege here is the only child in all of America to have this name. But what you have also done, most likely because you failed to do any research whatsoever on your made up word, is named your child a slang term for a geek or nerd (according to the Urban Dictionary). Why didn't you just name the kid Please Kick My Ass?

That one doesn't phase you? Your kid's going to be tough, right — he can handle that! Okay...I'll do you one better. I mean, did you think we were going to ignore the elephant in the room and NOT mention that your child's name is one of the most popular slang terms in the WORLD for a blowjob?

You actually named your child after a stiff, engorged penis ejaculating inside a hot, willing mouth. That's what you did. Of all the things in the world, that's what you picked to make people think of when they think of your son.

So long, Beege...we hardly knew ye…

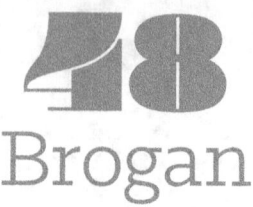

# Brogan

Ugh. Talk about a turd. I just said this name out loud and immediately upon hearing it I felt like someone had raped my ear.

I am guessing that Dad came up with this one. It sounds like something a man would do rather than a woman. I read that it's traditionally an Irish last name, although apparently they do use it as a first name over there as well. Cool. They also get drunk in the morning and are the masters of domestic assault — but I bet you probably wanted that for little Brogan too, huh?

If you want a tough name, go with Chuck. Or Mack. Or fucking anything but this shit. Here's an idea — give your kid a normal name so he doesn't have to be so tough all the time!

"Brogan" sounds like an experimental gay encounter between two straight dudes, fueled by excessive drinking and libido, and never spoken of again after the following morning.

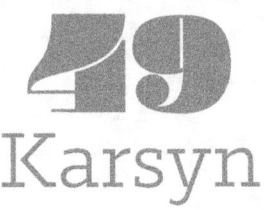

# Karsyn

Okay — now people are just fucking with me. They didn't *really* name a boy Carson, but then spell it like this. Please, dear God, tell me they didn't do that.

Turns out they did. In fact, they not only did they, then they went around submitting his picture to magazine contests. Poor little Karsyn's shittified name has been outed to the entire nation before he's even old enough to crawl.

I am truly baffled by this one. I am not a fan of the name Carson in the first place, but at least it's digestible. And he probably would have avoided torment if they had just spelled it like it's supposed to be spelled. They were so close to not shitting on this kid's life, then they went and laid a monster diarrhea all over it.

"Karsyn" sounds like a Danish exchange student with a perm.

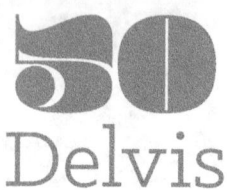

# Delvis

Un-fucking-believable.

I Googled this one and found it to be a lot more common than I would have EVER expected. Shit — more than one person with this atrocity is more common than I ever expected.

Who does this? Elvis is bad enough — but at least I know the reason behind it (even if it is an incredibly bad reason — naming your kid after some dead rock star that you wanted to suck off).

Delvis ranks right up there with Dilbert, Gomer and Uris as names you never, ever want to have.

All of those are better than Delvis, though. New candidate for the worst name ever.

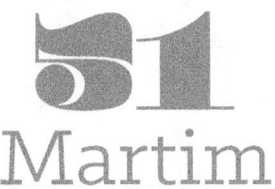

# Martim

There is only one reason to name a kid this, and that is to fuck with him and everyone else. That's it. No other reason exists.

You could very simply name him Martin, which is normal and sounds almost identical to Martim. You gain absolutely nothing by changing that last letter from "n" to "m."

But no — you had to fuck with all of us. Now he will spend the rest of his like correcting people. Don't you realize how fucking tedious this will become for Martim? EVERYONE will think it's an "n" at the end of his name. EVERYONE.

I hope you fuckers like sitting in your own shit and playing cribbage, because Martim's gonna put you bastards in a home the first chance he gets.

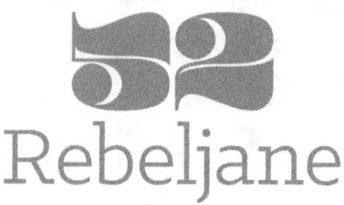

# Rebeljane

I actually saw this one attached to an adult who had passed away, but I had to include it because it just has to be on the all-time worst names list. It's all one word — Rebeljane.

On second thought, this may be the best name ever. I can't decide.

Obviously she wasn't that much of a fucking rebel, or she would've given a parents a big fuck-you by changing her name to something else.

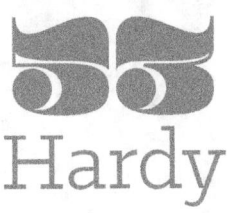

# Hardy

It's getting to the point that I think parents are just starting to mail it in. They hear a word that, at the time, sounds like a good word — then they name their kid with it.

Look, I like the word "orgasm." It makes me think good thoughts. I also love the word cocktail — it relaxes me. But I have the self-restraint not to name my daughter Orgasm Cocktail just because the words sound delightful rolling off my tongue.

And besides, Hardy is WAY too close to "hard-on" for me to ever consider fucking my son's life up with it.

Plus, the Hardy Boys were incestuous gay lovers and everyone fucking knows it.

# Journey

Here we go again. First we had a Boston, now a Journey. I guess I will have to save room in my next book of shitty names for Kansas, Triumph, Rush and Lynyrd Skynyrd.

It's obvious to me that people just don't say shit out loud before they go and stick a name on their kids. And don't give me that , "Oh, but it's beautiful" shit either. I'll prove it to you:

Have you ever had someone say to you,

> *Dude, I'm so stoked that 'Don't Stop*
> *Believein'' by Journey is popular again.*

and then you replied, "Did you say the word 'journey'? Wow — that sure is a beautiful word."? No, you fucking haven't.

Put down the glass pipe, Mom. This is a fucking horrible name for a child.

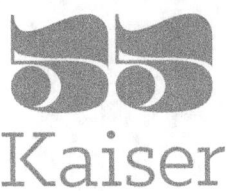

# Kaiser

Ummmm...okay. I guess if when the boy is born, he happens to be screaming, "Geben Sie mir einige Milch!" and the afterbirth is sauerkraut — then this would be an appropriate first name. Otherwise, it's scheisse.

Plus, if you're going to name your kids after a significant 19th century historical figure from the Prussian/Austro-Hungarian theater....DUDE, how could you overlook Otto von Bismarck or Archduke Franz Ferdinand? Christ, would you have drafted Sam Bowie over Michael Jordan, too? Ryan Leaf over Peyton Manning?

But I'm sure you already FUCKING knew that.

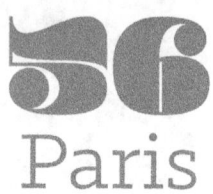

# Paris

I never thought I would have to criticize people for this grave naming error. I just figured the night vision boner suck-fest video - or the countless other brainless adventures of the heiress of the same name - would take care of this name on its own. Instead, I see it popping up now and again.

The bottom line is this — if you name your daughter Paris, she will be expected to be a dumb slut. Trust me on this one. And if she somehow manages NOT to be a slut, she will still be called one.

Oh, and your daughter will never go to Paris. She will almost certainly, however, be Eiffel Towered at one point. (Google it)

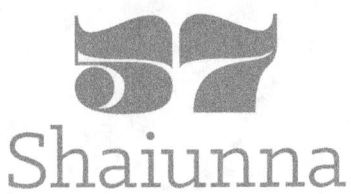

# Shaiunna

Here's a story that perfectly illustrates the kind of people that name their kids stupid shit like Shaiunna. This little girl was a 2 year old that I read about in the news. Notice I said "was" — turns out Mom's boyfriend kept a pet python in the house and, predictably, the python got out and strangled the child to death.

Sad story, to be sure. The moral of the story is this: if you are fucking dumb, don't have children.

If you have them, give them up for adoption — BEFORE you name them.

To this day, no one has ever pronounced Shaiunna's name correctly.

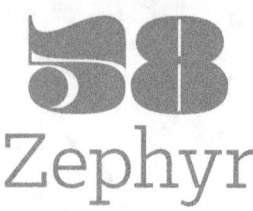

# Zephyr

I just saw this name on a list entitled "Old Fashioned Boy Names."

What the fuck? I have never once heard of anyone named Zephyr. If I did, I would be immediately compelled to kick his ass. That's the kind of natural reaction that normal, calm, rational people, such as myself, have to a name like this.

How old-fashioned are we talking? Sure, there may have been a mythological Greek character named Zephyr - and technically that would be old fashioned - but come on, people!

I say, if you're going the old-fashioned route, kick it up a notch. Cavemen were around way before the Greeks. Name your kid "UGGGH" or "Grrrr" or "Holy Fuck, Run, It's a Mastodon!"

C'mon, aren't you unique and creative enough?

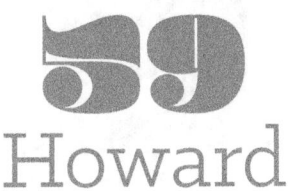

# Howard

Why would I fuck with this name? It's about as standard and classic as an American first name gets — for a boy. But I am talking about a girl named Howard. Howard Allen, in fact. Yeah - it's pretty bad.

Luckily for her, she had a lot more smarts than most kids, and on the first day of school she told her teacher that her name was Anne. Which, by the way, is fucking awesome and we love her for it. Five years old, and she's already stepping up to the plate and calling bullshit on her fucking nimrod parents.

Later on she got married, and the transition was complete — from Howard Allen O'Brien to Anne Rice. Yes, the best-selling author Anne Rice started out as Howard Allen O'Brien. She said her Mom wanted to name her after her father, and she thought it was unique.

And now, you know...the rest of the story...

She came through it okay, so this proves that you CAN name your kid something fucked up and he or she can still excel, right?

Wrong.

You see, not only is she much smarter than your future child (she has sold over 100 million books and is one of the best-selling authors of all-time), don't forget she sold every one of them with a *different* name.

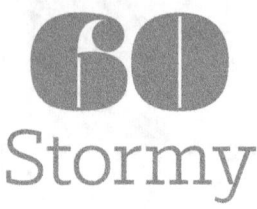

# Stormy

It saddens me that I have seen this name way more often that once. Not surprisingly, each time I have seen it, there was a mobile home lurking nearby. And inside the mobile home was a makeshift strip club, at which "Stormy" was the feature dancer. Because she was the only dancer. Because people named Stormy have no other option in life other than to become a self-employed stripper out of their own trailer.

You have it backwards, Mom and Dad. This is the name your daughter calls herself after she inevitably becomes a stripper, not one you give her before.

Now what's she going to call herself on the pole — Kathy?

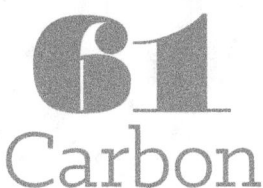

# Carbon

Unfuckingreal.

This one is most certainly the result of his parents being wrapped up in the global warming phenomenon. Why else would you name your kid after a nonmetallic and tetravalent chemical element?

Look — it's one thing to have a hard-on for a cause. Personally, I like dogs and think that adopting a rescue dog is one hell of a cool thing to do. But Jesus — I don't name my fucking kid Canine or Rin-Tin-Tin. Keep your hobbies separate from what you name your kids.

If this kid's middle name is Footprint, I hope he disowns his parents as soon is he is old enough, leaving them to die sad and full of regret. And if it isn't — I hope he does exactly the same thing — after he kicks the shit out of them.

Honestly, I hope the kid has a really great middle name that....wait for it... wait for it....OFFSETS his Carbon first name! Fuckin' RIM. SHOT.

Fuck you guys.

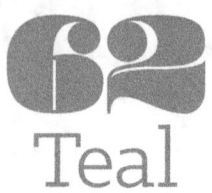

# Teal

Teal is a color, not a name. It's that blue-green color that was really, really common for a while — especially in cars, clothing for obese language-arts teachers and the waiting rooms of Asian massage parlors.

It got so common, in fact, it became overdone and after a while no one wanted a teal car anymore.

Interesting...I wonder of Teal's middle name, then, is McKenzie or Britney or some other overdone bag of waste? Probably not. It's probably Maroon, or Hunter Green, or Honda Del Sol.

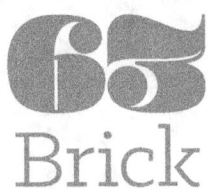

# Brick

Ahhh...the fail proof name, right? How could you go wrong with a powerful boy's name like Brick? Your boy is gonna be strong and confident and reliable! Strong as a brick, he'll be!

Yeah — unless he isn't. Then he's going to be mincemeat. If you have a name like Brick, you can bet your ass you are going to be challenged to a fight. And another, and another, and another.

Possibly worse yet is if you turn out to be an awkwardly skinny or overly plump guy. Then the name looks even more ridiculous on you that it would on someone of normal size or a big, strong guy.

The only reason to name a kid Brick is because you have your own inadequacies and you want so badly for your son to grow up strong and tough.

Remember — it's not about you, asshole. You didn't hit the big home run in high school. Get over it.

Oh, and of course, he'll never be called anything but Prick.

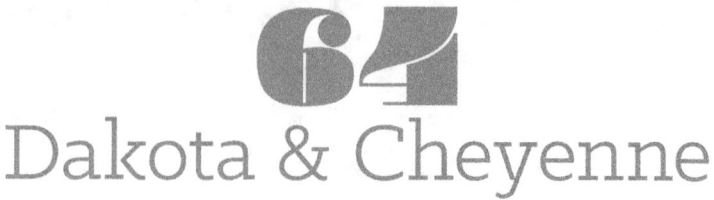

# Dakota & Cheyenne

You know — there sure are a lot of Dakotas and Cheyennes out there. Interesting, since Wyoming and the Dakotas are 3 of the bottom 5 states in terms of population. I think there are probably more people named Cheyenne than the actual population of Cheyenne itself.

Have you ever been to North Dakota or Wyoming? Of course you fucking haven't, because there's no reason to go there. It's freezing cold 9 months out of the goddamned year, everyone thinks fine dining is Applebee's and it's teeming with oil-rig hellraisers who spend their fat paychecks on methamphetamine and traveling hookers.

Your child is not a cowboy or cowgirl. He or she will not ride a bull or be a rodeo queen. Stop this bullshit infatuation with the West.

If you want to name your kid something that really mimics the spirit of the old West, name it Cholera, Smallpox or Opium Den.

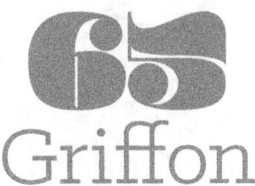

# Griffon

Pretty cute name for a boy, huh?

> *Hey Griffon, let's go toss the*
> *ol' pigskin around the back yard!*

That is, until you learn that it means either a type of wire haired hunting dog used to retrieve animals that have been blown to shit, or a type of vulture that feeds on the flesh of rotting animal carcasses, or that mythical lion-eagle cross-breed, which your child will never resemble, because he is actually crossbred with a male human who plays too much World of Warcraft and a female human with no self-esteem.

Do your research, assholes.

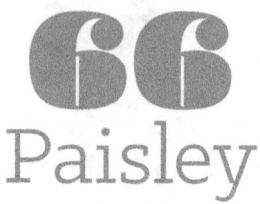

# Paisley

Delightful. You named your kid after a clothing pattern popular in the fuck-happy 60s. I guess we should all be glad that you didn't opt for Denim or Leisure Suit.

This poor gal will get every fucking thing on Earth made of Paisley as a gift throughout her life. "Happy birthday! Look — it's a paisley, stuffed cat that doubles as a draft blocker! I got it because it's paisley — and you're Paisley!"

I guess it's a good thing Paisley isn't a boy. He'd have a closet full of black & blue paisley ties — you know, to match the bruises on his face from getting his ass kicked for being named Paisley.

All of the above scenarios are preferable to the superlatively repulsive idea that the child could be named after country singer Brad Paisley, who is the most detestable living person on the planet.

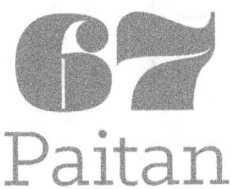

# Paitan

## Pie-tan? Payton? Pay-tan? Pie-ton?

How the fuck am I supposed to pronounce this one? Is it a normal name misspelled, or is it a brand new name? Does the name come with some sort of a hint or a clue — like maybe his middle name is something along the lines of Manning or MyFirstNameIsPronouncedPieTan?

There are just too many unanswered questions when you pull shit like this. I guarantee you that all of you reading this had no fucking idea how to pronounce this poor bastard's name when you read it either — and neither will people who matter, like potential employers.

But Mom and Dad know how, right? And that's all that matter to them — because little Paitan is different. And special. And doomed.

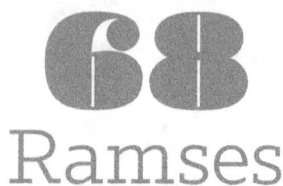

# Ramses

I admit — Ramses is a pretty strong sounding name. Ramses was a leader — a great Egyptian Pharaoh who is known for being strong yet sound. He was also known for settling differences with diplomacy rather than war, by entering into the first ever peace treaty.

Oh yeah — and Ramses is also known for being the name of a FUCKING BRAND OF CONDOMS! Jesus...I can think of few names that would do more damage to a kid than this one. Maybe Trojan. Possibly Jimmy Hat. Probably Dick Wrapper. But my point is, the list is very short.

I know, I know — but Mom & Dad named his after the great man, not the dong sheath. Do you think Mikey Williams in Ramses' 6th grade class gives a fuck how or why he got his name? Hell no! When the other kids figure out that there's a brand of condoms called Ramses, little darling here will be known as "Cock Sock" for the rest of his school days — which may be shorter than most if he can't take the abuse and drops out.

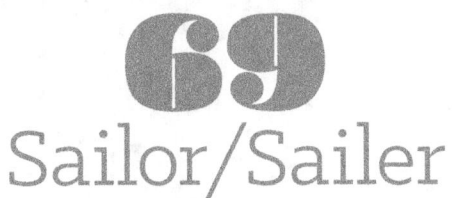

# Sailor/Sailer

I actually had someone propose that I name my very own child this ridiculous "name." That person is no longer in the circle of trust.

With "names" like this starting to pop up, it proves that people have gone beyond simple craziness, and are now just trying to see how far they can push the envelope before our government steps in and starts making laws to prevent this shit (I'm usually for smaller government, but I would give them a pass in the naming arena).

## Seriously...Sailor? Why not Marine? Or Seaman. Or Cum.

It doesn't even make sense within the lunatic world of stupid baby-naming. Sailing is a thing people do in their leisure time, or an occupation, if you're in the Navy. Is that what this is about? Like naming your kid Soldier or Serviceman? Or Welder?

I have no idea what's going on here.

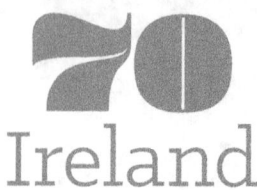

# Ireland

I have now seen this name more than once, so I feel compelled to add it to the book.

I believe these people were looking at Irish names because they like shitty Irish bar-music bands like The Pogues or Flogging Molly or Dropkick Murphys or whatever, and after passing on Seamus, Keegan and Dublin for being "not Irish enough," they said "fuck it all" and named their kid after the entire country. Well done, my retarded friends.

I have some German blood in me, I think I may name my kid Federal Republic of Germany. Or I might go with another country in the region, since FRG is probably overdone. Maybe Austria. Or Lichtenstein.

There is not a single country in existence that would work well as a name (except possibly Uzbekistan). Not even the good old U.S. of A. I knew a girl named America once — she suffered for it.

All of the Irelands will too.

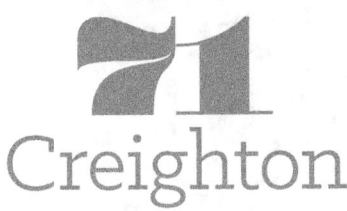

# Creighton

I looked this one up after I found it, and it said that Creighton is a "very rare male first name." No shit, huh? That's because it's also a "very popular surname." In other words, it's a last name, you fucks!

This is someone's attempt to be snooty. Maybe this name is common amongst the Winchesters, the Hiltons and other blue-bloods of the world. But the kid that I saw it attached to was, er...let's just say he was not a blue blood. In their defense, I'm really, really, really shocked they didn't spell it "Crayton" (but I'm sure someone else has).

I understand — it's very difficult to accept that you are not rich, and not even very successful for that matter. But naming your kid Creighton, Forbes or Whitworth will not only NOT make you rich, it will make them the target of all of the other kids who know that they are not rich.

If you want to pretend your kid is rich, just name him Rich.

# silence

Wishful thinking. I like the idea, but I don't think that it will give you a quiet, well-behaved child. Especially when she's constantly sobbing from the emotional abuse she's been made to endure at school.

And don't try reverse psychology and name her Noizy either — it will cause just as many problems.

I am, though, a little amused by the thought of some authority figure bellowing

## "SILENCE!"

and this poor little shit looking up and saying, "What?" every time.

If I was named Silence, I'd always tell the teacher it was a misprint and that my real name is Violence, which is way more badass.

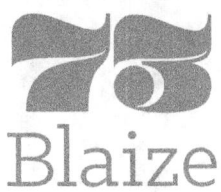

# Blaize

Here's another case of "look that shit up before you saddle your kid with it, idiots!" If little Blaize here was named before the internet and Google came along, I will give his parents a break (although the name still sounds like shit).

But in .11 seconds, a Google search reveals that the name Blaize means "lisp" or "stutter." So if the kid didn't have a natural speech impediment, he certainly will after the first couple of years of relentless taunting and torment from the other kids about his shitty name.

And, of course, there's that whole stoner thing. "420 BLAZE IT UP BRAH!" Sheesh…

If you like blazes, just set your trailer on fire for the insurance money and be done with it. No need to involve your kid.

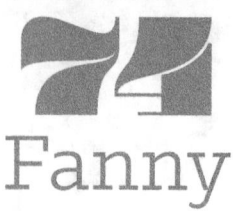

# Fanny

Here's a good example of an old name that used to be just fine and dandy to name your kid. Now it means ass. Use your head.

If it were me, I'd steer clear of Dick too. Just sayin'…

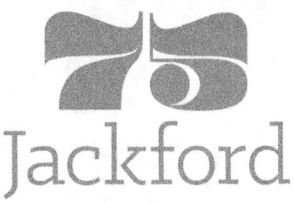

# Jackford

What the fuck is this now?

This is like some evil smash up of a first and last name, all crammed into one very awful first name.

I did a little research and found only ONE listing of this name in the entire United States. Congratulations, Mom & Dad!!!! You did it! You are so fucking clever you came up with a name that no one else had. Jackford's so special now, isn't he?

In case you have any more kids, here are a few suggestions of other first names that no one else in America has: Bobsanderson, Ericshackleford, Larryoreilly and Stevenmasterson.

Taser and beanbags for these shitheads, too.

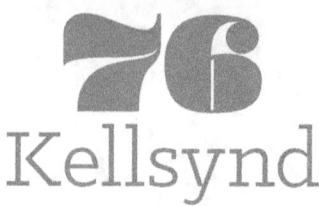

# Kellsynd

I couldn't find shit on this name, except that some horrible parents stuck in on her kid (presumably daughter, but you never know with these people).

I don't get what the appeal is of trying to name your child some name that no one else has ever had? You do realize that your name means shit to who you actually are, who you become?

Unless, of course, your name is some outlandish bullshit like Kellsynd, that causes you to get teased constantly and eventually turns you into a social recluse or a homicidal maniac.

Am I saying that Kellsynd will be a murderer? Yes. Yes I am. And it's all your fault, Mom and Dad.

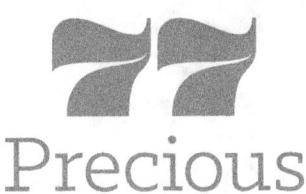

# Precious

News flash — we all think our little babies are precious. We just have the willpower not to name them that.

Know why? Because it's an adjective, not a name. And also because most other people — you know, those people that have to deal with our little darlings on a daily basis — they DON'T think Precious is all that precious.

Plus — how ridiculous does this name sound when Precious is an adult in the waiting room of the doctor's office? "Precious! Precious Jones!" Everyone in the waiting room will be embarrassed for her — but not half as much as she will be for herself.

Name your dog Precious. Name your kid something with some thought behind it.

*__Bonus:__ There was a movie called "Precious" about a girl named Precious. Precious weighed 400 pounds, got fucked by her stepfather and generally failed at everything in life.*

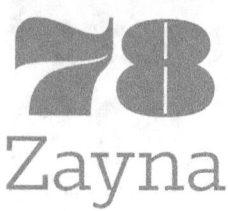

# Zayna

## All names beginning with the letter "Z" are shit.

Sure, there are a few exceptions to the rule, like Zachary and ummm, and... ummm, well, like Zachary. But that pretty much sums up the acceptable "Z" names.

If you have the uncontrollable urge to name your kid something that starts with the letter Z, please follow this simple plan — Step 1: Don't fucking name your kid anything that starts with the letter Z.

See? That was easy, boys and girls!

Exception: If you're from Eastern Europe, this doesn't apply to you, because we know every fucking third male name starts with a Z and usually has two or three additional Z's sprinkled in there before you hit the end of it.

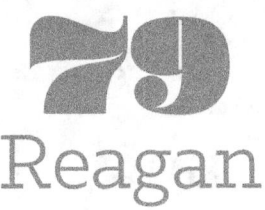

# Reagan

Please, I am begging you, PLEASE stop naming your daughters Reagan. It's not anywhere near as cute as you think it is. No matter how many of your Weight Watcher's buddies tell you it's "darling"...it's just not.

Yes, Reagan was a great President. But if you will recall correctly, he spent the last years of his life shitting himself and playing tic-tac-toe against a house fern. Not to mention the 2 most obvious facts — that Reagan was his *last* name...and that he was a fucking MAN!

And if you named her Reagan after something besides Ronald Reagan, well then...that's even more stupid.

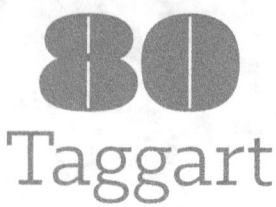

# Taggart

Wait a minute — isn't Taggart the last name of that super minister from Colorado that got caught rooting around in some other fella's butthole and smoking meth? I do believe it is. Too close for comfort if you ask me.

And even if this little guy was born before Ol' Ted started doing crank and fishing for brown trout — what kind of a first name is Taggart? Well, I looked it up and wouldn't you know — apparently it means "son of the priest." What are the odds?

And yeah, we know, Dagny Taggart from "Atlas Shrugged" by Ayn Rand is a libertarian icon. As a fellow Libertarian, to this I say: fuck you, still. Whether you're right, left or center, stop grafting your fucking political views onto your children.

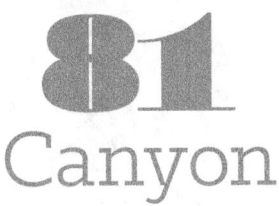

# Canyon

God, I hope this is not a little girl. Please tell me no one on this Earth would be cruel enough to stick that name on a little girl.

I refuse to even consider that to be an option, so a little boy it is. How could anyone possibly think this name sounded good? As much as I hate names like Piper and McKenzie and Hunter and the like — at least I can concede that they may have a small ring to them. Canyon? Not so much.

New rule — geological formations and related items should be avoided when naming your kids. The following are unacceptable: Canyon, Rock, Glacier, Gorge, Chasm, Quarry, Crevasse, Cave and Pangea. Cliff sucks too, but it's grandfathered in.

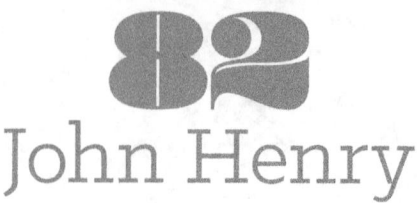

# John Henry

Standing alone, each of these names are traditional and just fine. But today I read about a kid that goes by John Henry. That's what the other kids call him. Not John, whose last name happens to be Henry. They say,

> *Hey, John Henry...wanna play?*

I am not certain, but I doubt that he's a large, black, steel-drivin' man.

Don't name your kids after legendary figures. I don't hear of many Paul Bunyans or Pecos Bills running around. Wanna know why? Because they're fucking stupid names. Just like John Henry.

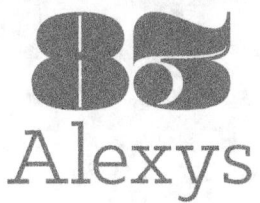

# Alexys

Complete slut. No way around it.

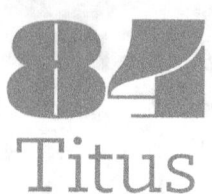

# Titus

What the fuck — did you give birth to a fucking Roman Emperor? I bet that brass helmet with the comb on top left a hellacious episiotomy scar, eh?

Mom and Dad really had to dig deep in the archives to pull this one out. Sure, he was a good emperor, I suppose...but so were Vespasian and Pertinax. You don't see little guys running around Jefferson Elementary with those names, do you? Wait — don't answer that. The way things are going these days, you probably do.

It's a special kind of tiny-dicked father who names his kid after emperors, but there's enough of them out there that you probably know one. Titus, Maximus, Caesar, Augustus, even Alexander (a fine name, but equally unacceptable if you're naming him after Alexander the Great, or even hoping that people start referring to your son that way, which makes you a pompous cunt).

Name your Great Dane Titus. Name your kid something less Flavian Dynasty-ish.

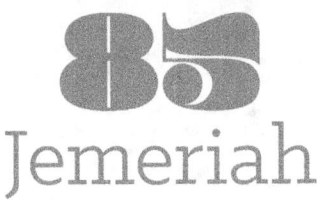

# Jemeriah

This is a new move on the part of Mom and Pops — one I hadn't seen before. I've seen the "add a letter", and the "replace one letter with a different, random letter." I've also seen the "intentional misspell." This one is the "juxtapose two letters in the name" bit. Clever...very clever indeed.

The problem is that the kid will undoubtedly be call Jeremiah 99% of the time, thus virtually destroying your little selfish work of art. Don't fuck with a perfectly good name. Just leave the letters in the order in which the Hebrews intended them to be.

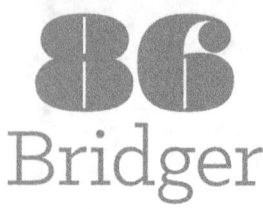

# Bridger

I got this "name" from a good friend of mine. He said he overheard the name at a garage sale. That figures. His folks were probably out shopping for more discount names.

Bridger is by far one of the worst names that I have heard. It makes no sense and came from nowhere.

Sometimes I seriously consider going back to college, getting an education degree, and then becoming a teacher, just so I can look parents like this in the eye and make sarcastic comments until the school board fires me. As in, "Bridger. Ah. Bridger. I see. (Very hard, slow, eye roll). Ohhhh kayyy…"

Maybe the little shit's dad builds bridges, but more likely the little shit's dad lives under one.

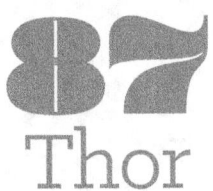

# Thor

Obviously, this is not a new or made up name, but it is stupid nonetheless.

If you can guarantee that your child is going to be a strapping, menacing Viking-like warrior with bulging muscles of stone and flowing, blonde locks — then Thor is fair game. If there is any chance at all that your kid will be anything less, then Thor is a curse.

By the way, I think a lot of people pronounce this "tore" and not "thor." That makes it infinitely worse.

Scandinavians, you're excluded from ridicule here, since I think your Thor is like our John Smith. Or, should I say, our Britney McKenzie Caden Keegan Aidan Smith.

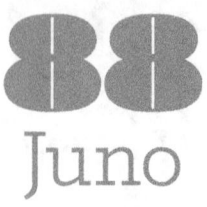

# Juno

This name is creeping up more and more these days, ever since that cutesy little movie of the same name came out a few years back. Good idea, people — name your kid after a movie character who's an apathetic teenaged girl dealing with an unplanned, unwanted pregnancy. If you're lucky, your very own little Juno will be knocked up by the time she's 11!

I know it's a Roman goddess, but don't act like you named her after the fucking Queen of the Gods, because that's bullshit.

One time when I was blackout hungover and getting breakfast at some shitty diner, this old man was eating behind us with his young granddaughter who was apparently named Juno. He kept saying "Juno want toast?" as a joke, but the kid wasn't catching on, so he kept saying it and pissing the kid off, like 40 times. I laughed so hard I almost vomited at the table.

Everyone will do this to everyone named Juno, until all of the little Junos want to die. Juno like that? Juno think so? Juno coming with us?

On second thought...please name your child Juno. All of you.

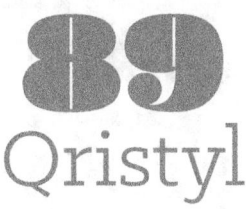

# Qristyl

There's just no excuse for shit like this. Hell, the name Crystal, spelled correctly, is bad enough. How many Crystal's have you met that live in a home that doesn't have wheels?

None...that's how many.

And then you go and spruce it up like this? Holy SHIT! Nothin' like sticking a candle in a turd and calling it a birthday cake.

"Qristyl" sounds like an artificial sweetener that gives you leukemia.

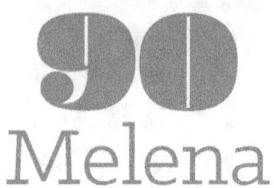

# Melena

What a pretty name. This is fairly benign, right? Not too crazy, not too "out there." It isn't spelled with seven Ms or eleven Ls. It doesn't spin off of a classic name with some new spelling or have letters added or subtracted. So...why in the hell did I add it?

Classic case of "do your research", folks. Just because it sounds pretty doesn't mean that it is. Far from it in this case. Melena is a medical term that refers to the "black, tarry feces that are associated with gastrointestinal hemorrhaging."

It's shit, people. Dark, black shit.

Yeah — let the kids on the playground get a hold of THAT little nugget of info.

# 91
# Huckleberry

Normally I would not have added this, since it's so far out there that I figured no one would really consider naming their kid Huckleberry. It's exactly why I have never mentioned that Penn Jilette (of Penn & Teller) has a daughter named Moxie Crimefighter or that Jason Lee has a kid named Pilot Inspektor. The names are awful, but I know that they will probably be the only people ever to have these names, so I didn't waste my breath.

Just this morning I saw TWO instances of kids named Huckleberry. Both of them called their kids "Huck."

If I could somehow relay to you in writing a shameful, lost look with incessant head shaking, I'd be doing it right now. Not only does Huck sound like a shoeless, overalls wearing, mouth breathing, wheat stalk chewing, backwards-assed little redneck hick who calls black people "niggers," — it also rhymes with "fuck."

Really, man? Nothing? None of this was considered as you put pen to paper in the delivery room?

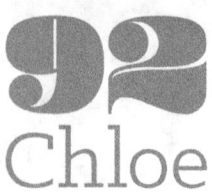

# Chloe

Enough with the Chloes already! It was kind of cute the first 10,000,000,000 times — now it's just as fucking worn out as McKenzie.

Not for nothing, it's also one of the most popular porn-star names in the entire adult industry. Among the audience of voracious online pornography consumers (read: everyone your child goes to school with), "Chloe" is synonymous with "that hot redhead whose eyes roll back to the whites when she cums and whose pussy can squirt across an entire living room." Yay!

Plus, it means "green shoot." What the fuck is that? Sounds like a bad case of V.D. to me.

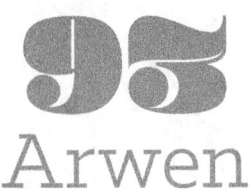

# Arwen

I had never seen this one before, so I had to look it up. Many of you nerds out there probably already know this (and you should be ashamed of yourselves) — Arwen is some elfen creature from the Lord of the Rings Nerd-a-thon.

Look — I realize that this is probably your favorite movie or book. I get that. Extremely nerdy, but I can live with it. But damn — you nerds, of all people, remember what it was like growing up as a geek — getting made fun of all the time and having your asses handed to you weekly. Why in the world would you damn your kid to that right off the bat?

Arwen, you have little chance of making through the school years without enduring a lot of verbal abuse. I hope you can rise above the torture that your dork parents have created for you.

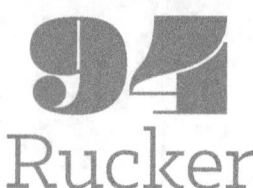

# Rucker

Where could this bastard name have come from? Darius Rucker is a good singer, but shit - he's not *that* good.

A better questions is, why am I still trying to get into these people's heads?

Never name your kid something that rhymes with "motherfucker." Or "cocksucker." He will never be called anything but those two things, by anyone.

Even his teachers. His teachers will refer to him as "Cocksucker," then pretend it was a slip of the tongue, and then call him "Cocksucker" again.

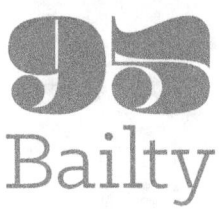

# Bailty

This is a wretched name standing alone — but what makes it worse is that the parents REALLY showed their asses in a national magazine. You see, not only did they name their child with arrogance and snobbery, they also submitted a picture of little Bailty all jezebelled up in full makeup at age 8 months.

You people make me sick.

We're getting close to the end here, so I'm just going to repeat this one more fucking time: Your children are not show pieces. They're not art projects, pets, or canvases on which you're obligated to ejaculate what you believe to be your creativity and uniqueness.

They aren't your property. They are little human beings. They are actual people.

Fuck you all.

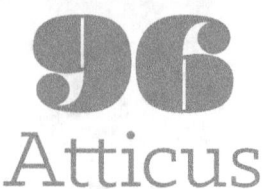

# Atticus

Come on! It's bad enough when people name their kids after present day movie characters like Benjamin Button and Wolverine — but Atticus? Seriously? Is his middle name Finch?

I bet Atticus is a tiny little bespectacled fella with a strong moral fiber. Either that, or he's a innocent kid that's about to endure a shit storm of teasing when he hits school age.

We get what's going on here. You want a throwback name, because everybody's all about throwin' back these days, yeah? Back when life was simpler. Folks talked to other folks. Everyone knew each other's name. The milkman brought nice fresh cold milk in glass bottles to your porch, and maybe even gave your old lady a pickle tickle now and then. Nowadays there's no civility or humanity or community. Everyone's glued to their phone or their computer and all the cars and restaurants and businesses are the same everywhere you go.

Fuck off already. Those were also the days where black people had their own drinking fountains, women weren't allowed to leave the kitchen, you could fingerbang your secretary right in the middle of the office and she would have to just sit there and giggle about it, doctors lit up a smoke while delivering babies, every car was death trap and you could do pretty much any crime and get away with it.

On balance, the past was shitty. No one should want to go back there, so stop fucking romanticizing it. And the stupid names that went along with it.

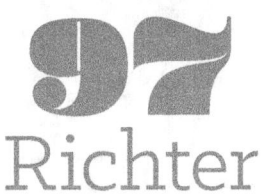

# Richter

I know I sound like a crotchety old man here (imagine that) — but what in the fuck has this world come to? Fucking Richter? As a first name?

I tried to research this, and shockingly the only place I found any reference to it as a first name was in one of those parenting rags. Their take on it was this,

> *A boy with this sharp-edged German name will cause seismic shocks wherever he goes.*

Fuckin-A right he will. Seismic shocks on his face and torso from the fists of the mean little bastards at his school.

Side note: Whose job is it to write those stupid little blurbs, and how badly does she want to kill herself every night? I bet she cuts herself with a razor blade just to feel something.

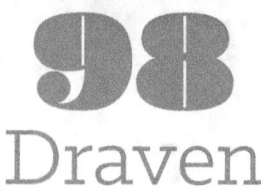

# Draven

Although this name is dreadful, I don't think the other kids will give him too much grief to his face. That's because his name makes him sound like a terrifying creature of the night. I was frightened to merely type it.

Instead, they will shun him, call him "Vampire Boy" and stay as far away from him as possible, for fear of Draven stealing their souls and making them blood kindred.

He'll live a lonely, nocturnal existence and hate you for it every time the sun comes up.

Weirdly enough, I'm getting the vibe that this is exactly the life his parents wanted for him.

All's well that ends well, I guess.

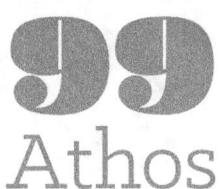

# Athos

One of the worst names yet, Athos is apparently a character in some Three Musketeers novel or some shit. According to the descriptions I read, Athos was a father figure to the other Musketeers, as well as a closet alcoholic.

Good work, Mom & Dad! Not only did you name your kid after a fictional character in some book because you thought it "sounded cool," you picked a drunken pedophile. Snazzy!

You two are both...Athos. Get it? Like, assholes? RIM. FUCKING. SHOT.

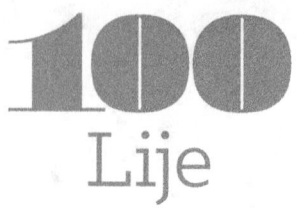

# Lije

Here we go again. Is it pronounced...

Lidge? Lie-Gee? Lee-hee? Lee-hay? Lie-hee? Litch? Is the "j" silent possibly, so his name his "Lie?"

Is there some sort of chart or legend to assist me? Can someone fucking help me out here?

I hope that the above scenario happens to Lije every single time a teacher, nurse, potential employer or anyone else tries to call out his name. Maybe after a certain number of times, he will get mad enough to kick the shit out of his parents for such ridiculousness.

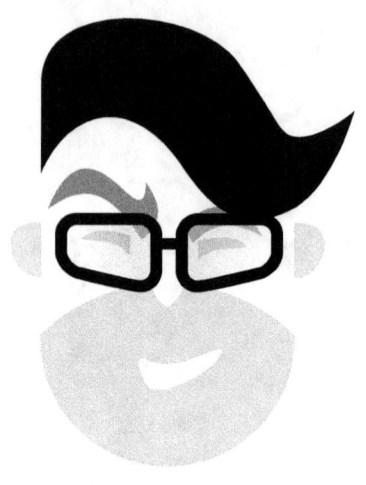

Thanks for reading. Now you're ready for volume two of our six books. If you were holding your breath hoping not to see your child's name here, don't worry — you can be nervous all over again with the next book. Believe me, these shithole names are NOT in short supply.

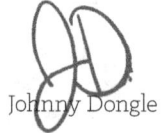

Johnny Dongle